Contents

KT-514-578

For the attention of the learner

You are not allowed to copy any information from this book and use it as your own evidence. That would count as plagiarism, which is taken very seriously and may result in disqualification. If you are in any doubt at all please speak to your teacher.

Acknowledgments

Photo credits

The authors and publishers would like to thank the following for permission to reproduce material in this book:

Page 17 © Misha – Fotolia.com; page 18 © Monkey Business – Fotolia.com; page 19 © By Ian Miles-Flashpoint Pictures / Alamy; page 20 © Art Directors & TRIP / Alamy; page 22 (top) © Andres Rodriguez – Fotolia.com; (bottom) © soundsnaps – Fotolia.com; page 24 © Peter Jordan / Alamy; page 25 © Noam Armonn / Alamy; page 26 © deanm1974 – Fotolia.com.

Every effort has been made to trace and acknowledge ownership of copyright. The publishers will be happy to make suitable arrangements with any copyright holders whom it has not been possible to contact.

BTEC

Level 2

HEALTH AND SOCIAL CARE

ASSESSMENT GUIDE

Unit 7 EQUALITY AND DIVERSITY IN HEALTH AND SOCIAL CARE

ELIZABETH RASHEED

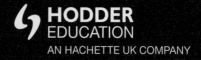

HODDER EDUCATION
AN HACHETTE UK COMPANY

The sample learner answers provided in this assessment guide are intended to give guidance on how a learner might approach generating evidence for each assessment criterion. Answers do not necessarily include all of the evidence required to meet each assessment criterion. Assessor comments intend to highlight how sample answers might be improved to help learners meet the requirements of the grading criterion but are provided as a guide only. Sample answers and assessor guidance have not been verified by Edexcel and any information provided in this guide should not replace your own internal verification process.

Any work submitted as evidence for assessment for this unit must be the learner's own. Submitting as evidence, in whole or in part, any material taken from this guide will be regarded as plagiarism. Hodder Education accepts no responsibility for learners plagiarising work from this guide that does or does not meet the assessment criteria.

The sample assignment briefs are provided as a guide to how you might assess the evidence required for all or part of the internal assessment of this Unit. They have not been verified or endorsed by Edexcel and should be internally verified through your own Lead Internal Verifier as with any other assignment briefs, and/or checked through the BTEC assignment checking service.

Orders: please contact Bookpoint Ltd, 130 Milton Park, Abingdon, Oxon OX14 4SB. Telephone: +44 (0)1235 827720. Fax: +44 (0)1235 400454. Lines are open from 9.00 a.m. to 5.00 p.m., Monday to Saturday, with a 24-hour message answering service. You can also order through our website www.hoddereducation.co.uk

If you have any comments to make about this, or any of our other titles, please send them to educationenquiries@hodder.co.uk

British Library Cataloguing in Publication Data

A catalogue record for this title is available from the British Library

ISBN: 978 1 444 1 8983 4

Published 2013

Impression number   10 9 8 7 6 5 4 3 2 1

Year   2016 2015 2014 2013

Copyright © 2013 Elizabeth Rasheed

Cover photo © Image Source / Alamy

Typeset by Integra Software Services Pvt. Ltd., Pondicherry, India.

Printed in Dubai for Hodder Education,
an Hachette UK Company,
338 Euston Road,
London NW1 3BH

Command words

You will find some of the following command words in the assessment criteria for each unit.

Analyse	Identify the factors that apply and state how these are related. Explain the importance of each one.
Assess	Give careful consideration to all the factors or events that apply and identify which are the most important or relevant.
Describe	Give a clear description that includes all the relevant features – think of it as 'painting a picture with words'.
Discuss	Consider different aspects of a topic and how they interrelate, and the extent to which they are important.
Evaluate	Bring together all the information and review it to form a conclusion. Give evidence for each of your views or statements.
Explain	Provide details and give reasons and/or evidence to support the arguments being made. Start by introducing the topic then give the 'how' or 'why'.
Summarise	Demonstrate an understanding of the key facts, and if possible illustrate with relevant examples.

UNIT 7
Equality and Diversity in Health and Social Care

Unit 7: Equality and Diversity in Health and Social Care is an internally assessed, optional, specialist unit with two learning aims:

- Learning aim A: Understand the importance of non-discriminatory practice in health and social care.
- Learning aim B: Explore how health and social care practices can promote equality and diversity.

The unit explores issues around delivering health and social care fairly in a culturally diverse society. We explore what is meant by discriminatory practice and its impact on service users and those giving care. We also look at how health and social care can be delivered in a way that does not discriminate and that meets individual needs and we look at the impact of such care.

Learning aim A explores the importance of having health and social care practices that do not discriminate.

Learning aim B explores how we can encourage equality and diversity through the way we deliver health and social care.

Each learning aim is divided into two sections. The first section focuses on the content of the learning aim and each of the topics is covered. At the end of each section there are some knowledge recap questions to test your understanding of the subject. The answers for the knowledge recap questions can be found at the end of the guide.

The second section of each learning aim provides support with assessment by using evidence generated by a student, for each grading criterion, with feedback from an assessor. The assessor has highlighted where the evidence is sufficient to satisfy the grading criterion and provided developmental feedback when additional work is required.

At the end of the guide are examples of assignment briefs for this unit. There is a sample assignment for each learning aim, and the tasks allow you to generate the evidence needed to meet all the assessment criteria in the unit.

Learning aim A

Understand the importance of non-discriminatory practice in health and social care

Assessment criteria

2A.P1 Describe non-discriminatory and discriminatory practice in health and social care, using examples.

2A.P2 Describe how codes of practice and legislation promote non-discriminatory practice in health and social care.

2A.M1 Explain the importance of legislation and codes of practice in promoting non-discriminatory practice in health and social care, using examples.

2A.D1 Assess the impact of discriminatory practice for health and social care workers, with reference to selected examples.

Discriminatory and non-discriminatory practice in health and social care

Definition of non-discriminatory practice in health and social care

Studied

Non-discriminatory practice means:

- not treating any individuals or groups less fairly than others, which means we should treat all individuals and groups fairly
- valuing diversity, seeing differences as a positive thing
- adapting care to meet diverse needs.

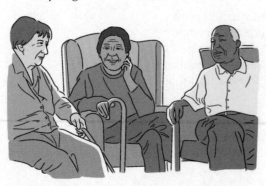

Figure 1.1 Care should be adapted to meet diverse needs

Examples of discrimination (bad practice) in health and social care

Studied ☐

- **Prejudice or 'prejudging' someone.** A very healthy 80-year-old lady wishes to donate a kidney but her donation is refused because she is too old. She is prejudged, discriminated against because of her age.
- **Stereotyping.** Having a fixed generalised belief about a group of people; for example, a belief that only teenagers sleep around so health campaigns about sexually transmitted infections are aimed only at them.
- **Labelling.** Seeing just one aspect and putting someone in a category; for example when people with partial sight are labelled as visually impaired and offered the same care as someone with no sight.
- **Refusing medical treatment.** This happens when older people are told that nothing can be done for them but in fact treatments are available but are only offered to younger people.
- **Offering inappropriate treatment or care.** This is discriminatory practice. People with dementia require specialist care, yet often they are placed in a care home where workers do not understand their needs.
- **Giving less time when caring for an individual than needed.** Staff cuts meant that on a ward with 32 patients who wet the beds, there were only two staff, so they could not give each patient the time needed to care for them properly.

Examples of non-discriminatory (good) practice in health and social care

Studied ☐

- **Providing appropriate health and social care to meet the needs of individuals**, such as large print leaflets for partially sighted people.
- **Adapting care to meet the diverse needs of different individuals**, such as offering relationship counselling to all, whether they are in a same-sex relationship or any other type of relationship.
- **Providing equality of access to health and social care services**, for example, by the personalisation of care, especially in the area of learning disabilities. Personalisation of social care puts the individual at the centre of the assessment process, so they can say what they need and make their own choices. This is done through:
  - person-centred planning
  - supporting people towards independent living
  - direct payments to the individual, so they can employ their own personal assistant.

Impact of discriminatory and non-discriminatory practice in health and social care

The effects of discrimination (bad practice) on service users

Studied ▢

These include:

- loss of self-esteem
- stress
- reluctance to seek support and treatment
- longer waiting times for some groups.

A 70-year-old person who is told they are too old to be treated will experience stress and a loss of self-esteem.

If signs and directions are small and difficult to read, someone with a visual impairment may find it stressful to attend a hospital appointment.

An alcoholic person may be reluctant to seek medical help for other problems because the doctor does not approve of her behaviour. A pregnant woman who does not speak English may be reluctant to seek advice from a doctor or midwife and may miss vital antenatal care.

Cuts to healthcare funding mean there are longer waiting times for some operations, such as joint replacement. Making people wait longer for their operations implies that their health is less important.

Non-discriminatory (good) practice meeting the diverse needs of individuals

Studied ▢

Non-discriminatory practice enables people to stay healthy and active. The 70-year-old person who is treated promptly will be back doing his voluntary work and leading an active and independent life.

Clear signage will enable a partially sighted person to get around the hospital independently.

A person who is treated without being prejudged is more likely to give up addictions than one who is condemned. A pregnant woman who does not speak English is more likely to attend an antenatal clinic if one of the care workers tries to speak a few words of the woman's language.

If a person is treated promptly they feel valued as a person, but equally important is that they can then get back to their normal life and be a productive member of society.

The importance of meeting legal and workplace requirements

Studied ☐

There are several laws and regulations that affect the workplace, for example:

- The Health and Safety at Work Act 1974, Manual Handling Operation Regulations 1992 (amended 2002), Data Protection Act 1998 and the Freedom of Information Act 2000. All cover aspects of equality but the law which focuses specifically on equality is the Equality Act 2010.
- The Equality Act 2010 protects people from discrimination, harassment and victimisation on the grounds of:
  - age
  - disability
  - gender reassignment
  - marriage and civil partnership
  - pregnancy and maternity
  - race
  - religion or belief
  - sex
  - sexual orientation.

Employers cannot discriminate on these grounds when employing people such as care workers and must make reasonable adjustments to help the person do the job. The law is meant to increase equality of opportunity for these groups. If an employer breaks this law they can be called before a tribunal, or in some cases taken to court.

Importance of following workplace and national codes of practice on non-discriminatory practice

A code of conduct for employers of social care workers and one for social care workers was published by the General Social Care Council. Both codes explain how to work in a way that does not discriminate against service users or workers.

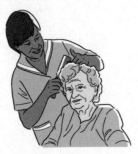

Figure 1.2 Social care workers must work to a code of conduct

- Employers must provide equal opportunity policies and procedures for service users and for staff.
- Social care workers must not discriminate or be prejudiced when working with service users or other co-workers.
- An employer or a social care worker who ignores the codes can be reported and disciplinary action may be taken if discrimination is proved. A social care worker may be removed from the professional register, and an employer ignoring the code may face sanctions.

As of 1 August 2012, the regulation of the social work profession and education transferred to the Health and Care Professions Council (HCPC) and the General Social Care Council (GSCC) closed. The codes of conduct are housed by Skills for Care.

The Nursing and Midwifery Council (NMC) has a code of conduct for professional nurses and midwives.

The NMC disciplinary process is similar to that of social care, with a regulatory body that holds conduct hearings. A nurse or midwife who is shown to be discriminatory may lose their registration, which means they cannot work as a nurse or midwife.

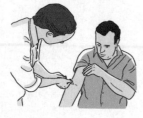

Figure 1.3 Nurses must also follow their own code of conduct

How legislation and codes of practice support non-discriminatory practice in health and social care

Studied ☐

Legislation and codes of practice make it a duty to be non-discriminatory. The legal framework:

- protects carers and service users
- enforces non-discriminatory practices
- enforces employer and employee responsibilities and ensures those who break the law face losing their registration
- ensures safeguarding.

Policies and procedures in the workplace help workers to be non-discriminatory.

If a care worker does discriminate, there is a complaints procedure and the care worker can be reported to their professional body.

Employers and employees each have a responsibility in this area – the employer must provide guidance and the employee must follow both it and their professional code.

Social workers, nurses, midwives and doctors can be reported to their regulatory body. If a conduct hearing finds them guilty, they may be de-registered, which means they can no longer work in that profession.

Both legislation and codes of practice work together to safeguard and protect all service users.

Knowledge recap questions

1. What does 'non-discriminatory practice' mean?
2. 'Giving less time when caring for an individual than needed' is an example of which type of practice?
3. Providing large print leaflets for partially sighted people is an example of what type of practice?
4. Give four effects of discrimination (bad practice) on service users.
5. The Equality Act 2010 protects people from discrimination, harassment and victimisation on which grounds?
6. Give three codes of practice or conduct relevant to health and social care workers.

Learning aim A: Understand the importance of non-discriminatory practice in health and social care

7

Assessment guidance for Learning aim A

Scenario

You have been volunteering at your local hospital, City Central, which takes patients from a wide range of different communities across the city. The volunteer coordinator knows you are studying health and social care and has asked you to produce a booklet to help new volunteers understand the importance of non-discriminatory practice. She has asked you to include a section on how codes of practice and legislation improve health and social care.

Include the following and give examples for each:
- A description of non-discriminatory and discriminatory practice
- A description of how codes of practice and current and relevant legislation promote non-discriminatory practice, explaining their importance in promoting non-discriminatory practice
- An assessment of the potential impact of discriminatory practice for health and social care workers.

2A.P1 Describe non-discriminatory and discriminatory practice in health and social care, using examples

Assessor report: The command verb in the grading criteria is **describe**. Learners should give a clear description of discriminatory and non-discriminatory practices. To illustrate their understanding, they should give examples of non-discriminatory or discriminatory practices for three of these categories:

- Examples of discrimination in health and social care, e.g. prejudice, stereotyping, labelling, refusal of medical treatment, offering inappropriate treatment or care, giving less time when caring for an individual than needed.

- Examples of non-discriminatory practice in health and social care, e.g. providing appropriate health and social care to meet the needs of individuals, adapting care to meet the diverse needs of different individuals, providing equality of access of health and social care services.

Learner answer

Discrimination in health and social care includes prejudice, stereotyping, labelling, refusal of medical treatment, offering inappropriate treatment or care, and giving less time when caring for an individual than needed. It means not treating people fairly **(a)**.

Non-discriminatory practice in health and social care includes providing the right care to meet the needs of individuals, adapting care to meet the different needs of different individuals, and making sure that everyone has the same access to health and social care services. It means treating people fairly, which is what we should do **(b)**.

Assessor report: The learner has made a good start by describing non-discriminatory **(b)** and discriminatory **(a)** practice in health and social care. They will now need to provide examples of each.

 Learner answer

Here are some examples of non-discriminatory and discriminatory practice **(c)**:

Jon has a problem with alcohol. He lives alone and does not take care of himself. One winter he has a very bad cold and has difficulty breathing. His neighbour persuades him to go to the doctor but when Jon goes to the surgery, the receptionist is very rude to him and tells him that they do not make appointments for drunks. This is an example of discriminatory practice.

Sumeyah is five months pregnant and has recently arrived in England to join her husband. She understands English but has not got confidence to speak it. At the antenatal clinic, the midwife explains everything slowly and uses pictures to help Sumeyah understand what checks are made. The midwife also gives her a leaflet in English and in Sumeyah's own language so that Sumeyah can take it home and discuss it with her husband. This is making sure that everyone has the same access to services and is non-discriminatory practice.

Assessor report: The learner has provided one good example of discriminatory and one good example of non-discriminatory practice **(c)**.

Assessor report – overall

What is good about this assessment evidence?

The learner included all the categories of discriminatory **(a)** and non-discriminatory **(b)** practice and has given two examples **(c)**, explaining what type of practice they show.

What could be improved about this assessment evidence?

In order to achieve 2A.P1, the learner should give another example of either discriminatory or non-discriminatory practice.

2A.P2 Describe how codes of practice and legislation promote non-discriminatory practice in health and social care

Assessor report: The command verb in the grading criteria is describe. Learners should give a clear description of at least two codes of practice and describe the ways in which these promote non-discriminatory practice in health and social care. Codes of practice may be relevant to either social care or health practitioners and should be the current versions of the codes. Learners do not need to know the complex details of these codes. Legislation should focus on the Equality Act 2010.

✍ Learner answer

Codes of practice and laws or legislation show people what is non-discriminatory practice in health and social care. Codes of practice guide professional people, telling them what they must do. Legislation or laws tell everybody, not just professionals, what they must do.

Nurses and midwives have a code of conduct set by the Nursing and Midwifery Council. It says they must treat people with dignity and treat them as individuals. Professionals cannot prejudge individuals or refuse to treat them because they do not like them or do not approve of their lifestyles. They cannot refuse to treat a drug addict for a broken leg, just because he or she is a drug addict. Professionals must treat everyone equally in their professional work. If they do not, they can be reported to the council for their profession, which will investigate what happened. Professionals such as doctors, nurses, and midwives who break their professional code of conduct may be taken off the register, which means they cannot work in the profession **(a)**.

Assessor report: The learner has described what codes of practice and legislation are, and has given one example of a code of practice, describing how it promotes non-discriminatory practice in health and social care **(a)**.

✎ Learner answer

Laws apply to everybody, not just professionals. The Equality Act 2010 protects people from discrimination, harassment and victimisation on the grounds of age, disability, gender reassignment, marriage and civil partnership, pregnancy and maternity, race, religion or belief, sex and sexual orientation. Employers cannot discriminate against people on these grounds, so this means everyone has a chance to be treated equally. Public bodies such as health care cannot discriminate so they cannot refuse to treat a person on the grounds of the categories in the Act; for example, they cannot refuse to give a person with learning disabilities advice on sexual health **(b)**.

Laws and codes of practice safeguard and protect everyone who uses health and social care services.

Assessor report: The learner has given a good description of how legislation (The Equality Act) promotes non-discriminatory practice.

Assessor report – overall

What is good about this assessment evidence?

The learner has given a good example of how a code of conduct regulates professional behaviour and stops discrimination **(a)**. They have also explained how legislation protects people from discrimination **(b)**.

What could be improved about this assessment evidence?

The learner should expand on this answer by including a description of how an additional code of practice promotes non-discriminatory practice, as described in the guidance.

Explain the importance of legislation and codes of practice in promoting non-discriminatory practice in health and social care, using examples

Assessor report: The command verb in the grading criteria is **explain**. Learners will need to extend the work they have provided for 2A.P1 and 2A.P2 to explain the importance of non-discriminatory practice in health and social care, using at least two relevant examples. The learner should use current and relevant legislation and codes of practice and explain how these promote non-discriminatory practice. Examples may be either of non-discriminatory practice, or discriminatory practices, highlighting the respective benefits or negative consequences of each.

✍ **Learner answer**

Non-discriminatory practice is important in health and social care because everyone at some time needs these services and they should be able to get them. The Equality Act 2010 says that services such as health and care should not discriminate against people and should not victimise or harass them. The code of conduct for nurses and midwives also says that they should not discriminate.

Here is an example: Mrs J married in her late forties and thought it was too late for her to have a baby. She was very happy to discover that after two years of marriage she was in fact pregnant. She went to the clinic for her antenatal care. The midwife she saw was very abrupt and told Mrs J that she was much too old to be having a baby, that there might be problems with the baby and she should think of having a termination while there was time. Mrs J left the clinic in tears. Later she decided to report the midwife to the Nursing and Midwifery Council.

This is an example of discriminatory practice on the grounds of age. It shows prejudice, and also offering inappropriate treatment. Mrs J wanted her baby and did not want to get rid of it. The midwife should treat every person equally and not discriminate against Mrs J just because she is older than most women having their first baby. This discrimination breaks the code of practice and the Equality Act. It has negative effects on Mrs J as she feels she is of less value than a younger woman, and it affects her self-esteem. As well as loss of self-esteem and causing her stress, it makes her reluctant to go to the clinic again.

Assessor report: The learner has made a good start by describing the importance of legislation and codes of practice in promoting non-discriminatory practice in health and social care, using an example.

Assessor report – overall

What is good about this assessment evidence?

The learner includes a code of practice and the Equality Act and gives an example of discriminatory practice, showing the negative effects of this.

What could be improved about this assessment evidence?

The learner should give a second example, either of non-discriminatory practice, or discriminatory practices, highlighting the respective benefits or negative consequences of the practice. It would be good to give an example from a different sector of health and social care to show that the learner understands the breadth of this sector.

2A.D1 Assess the impact of discriminatory practice for health and social care workers, with reference to selected examples

Assessor report: The command verb in the grading criteria is **assess**. Developing the two examples from 2A.M1, learners should give careful consideration to the impact of discriminatory practice for health and social care workers.

✍ Learner answer

> The impact of discriminatory practice for the midwife discussed in 2A.M1 was that – as a result of Mrs J's complaint – she was called before a disciplinary hearing of the Nursing and Midwifery Council. Other people had heard what she said and came forward as witnesses. It was proved that the midwife was discriminatory in her practice and as a result the disciplinary council decided to suspend her from practice for six months. This meant she could not work as a midwife for that period of time. As a result of this, her employer dismissed her.
>
> Mrs J could have taken her to court under the Equality Act but chose not to do so as she thought the professional body had disciplined the midwife enough.

Assessor report: The learner has made a good start in assessing the impact of discriminatory practice for this health worker.

Assessor report – overall

What is good about this assessment evidence?

The learner found out what would happen in this situation and explained the consequences for the midwife.

What could be improved about this assessment evidence?

Another example is required, preferably from a different area of care. It would be good to see an overall summary of the impact of discriminatory practice for health and social care workers in terms of deterioration of care practice and poor quality care becoming the normal thing.

Learning aim B

Explore how health and social care practices can promote equality and diversity

Assessment criteria

2B.P3 — Describe the different needs of service users in health and social care, with reference to examples.

2B.P4 — Describe how health and social care provision can be adapted to meet the diverse needs of different individuals, with reference to examples.

2B.M2 — Explain the benefits of adapting health and social care provision to meet the diverse needs of different individuals, with reference to two selected examples.

2B.D2 — Assess the effectiveness of health and social care provision for different individuals with diverse needs, with reference to two selected examples.

Factors that may affect the care needs of individuals

Gender

Studied ☐

A person's gender may affect their care needs. They may prefer a same-sex ward. Mrs X, admitted to a medical ward, is put in a room with three male patients, causing stress for her and the other patients.

Sexual orientation

Studied ☐

An individual's sexual orientation may affect their care needs. Mary Smith and her partner Sandy have been in a relationship for many years. When Mary has a stroke, only next of kin are allowed to visit, but as the hospital policy is to respect sexual orientation Sandy is allowed to visit. This helps Mary to relax and make a speedier recovery.

Gender reassignment

Studied

Toni has decided after counselling to change gender and become female. The nurse admitting Toni asks how she would like to be addressed. Using the correct form of address and respecting Toni's gender will positively influence care and recovery.

Age

Studied

Age affects care. Older patients in hospital may prefer a formal approach to care, being addressed as Mr or Mrs, but it is important to ask the individual what they prefer. Some like to be addressed by their first name.

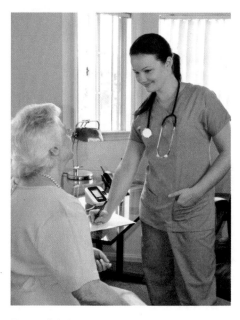

Figure 2.1 An older patient may prefer a more formal approach to care

Disability

Studied

Disability may affect care needs. A person with learning disabilities may find it difficult to get advice on having a baby. Someone with visual impairment may have difficulty finding out what services are available at their medical centre. Equality of access to services may be affected by disability.

Learning aim B: Explore how health and social care practices can promote equality and diversity

Marriage

Studied ☐

Marriage and civil partnership can affect care needs. We already saw that Mary Smith's wishes were respected by having her partner visit and this improved her chances of recovery. Sometimes people do not want the involvement of partners or family in their care. Their wishes must also be respected.

Pregnancy and maternity

Studied ☐

During pregnancy women are given a choice of birthing plan, including the type of delivery they would like, whether a home birth or hospital birth. They can choose who will be their birthing partner. During antenatal care they are offered advice about breastfeeding. If this advice is given in a way the person can understand, these factors positively affect how a woman copes with pregnancy and giving birth.

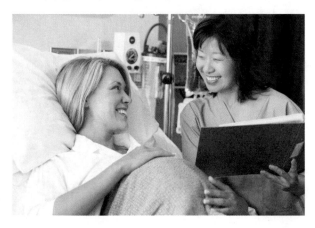

Figure 2.2 Giving good advice can positively affect how a woman copes with pregnancy

Race

Studied ☐

Race is a factor which should not affect access to services but unfortunately it does. Regardless of ethnic or national origins, people should be cared for according to their needs. However research shows that black and minority ethnic groups generally have worse health than other ethnic groups, and may be more likely to be diagnosed with mental health issues than other groups. Attempts are being made to change this.

Religion and belief

Religion and belief may affect the care needs of individuals.

Jehovah's Witnesses

Jehovah's Witnesses do not accept blood transfusions, so may not be able to have a vital operation. This can be an issue when children need treatment.

Judaism, Islam and Christianity – the Abrahamic religions

Festivals and holy days move according to the lunar calendar for the Christian festival of Easter and the Muslim festival of Eid. Fasting – going without food – or special food may be needed at that time.

The Jewish Passover requires special food, eaten in a specific order. Relatives may bring in food so the person can share the festival ceremony but if the person is in hospital prepared for theatre this may be a problem. Muslims fast during Ramadan, not eating or drinking anything between sunrise and sunset. This may affect their care if they are diabetic, as they will need to adjust their insulin and eating times to after sunset. Neither Jews nor Muslims eat pork, and both require that any meat should be killed in a special way. Jews call this *kosher* and Muslims call this *halal*. If this is unavailable, both Jews and Muslims may require vegetarian food.

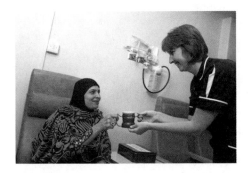

Figure 2.3 A Muslim may have special dietary requirements

In these religions communal prayer is important, but when someone is unable to attend a place of worship they can pray alone. Strict Muslims pray five times a day facing Mecca. Jews pray three times a day.

Symbols such as a cross, crescent or Star of David may help religious people cope with illness. A patient in hospital, or a resident in a care home, may like to keep a copy of the Bible with them if they are Christian, a copy of the Koran if they are Muslim or a copy of the Torah if they are Jewish.

Learning aim B: Explore how health and social care practices can promote equality and diversity

Hinduism and Buddhism

Hinduism is closely linked with Jainism, Buddhism and Sikhism. Most Hindus are vegetarian and even those who eat meat will not eat beef. Some Buddhists and some Sikhs are vegetarian too. Some people are vegan, which means they do not eat any animal products such as eggs or milk products.

Forms of worship vary. Many Hindus have a small shrine at home where they pray and offer a flower to the deity. Buddhists may use meditation.

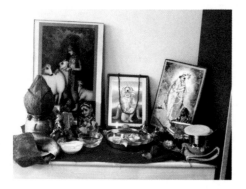

Figure 2.4 Hindus may have a small shrine at home

Secular groups

Secular beliefs must be respected. An atheist who does not believe in God or a humanist who aims to make the best of life whether there is a God or not, must have their views respected. Many secular people who do not have a religion use meditation to help them cope with illness. Usually, religious care needs are met in hospital by providing a quiet room where people of all religions or no religion can find peace.

The end of life is a time when people may turn to religion or may wish to talk to a religious person such as a priest. The important thing is to ask the person you are caring for what their religious needs are, and not make assumptions. It is important to respect the care needs of individuals and not to impose other religious beliefs on people. Christians, Muslims, Jews, Hindus and Buddhists believe there is life after death, and this may bring comfort when they are at the end of life. They may wish to visit their place of worship or have a person visit them. Many Catholics would like to make a confession before they die. It is very important to find out what the person wants and not make assumptions. Just because a person is Catholic, it does not mean they will wish to talk to a priest.

Social class

Studied ▢

Social class affects whether people have access to health care. A professional person is likely to have better education, housing and a better diet, and therefore better health. They know how to get services.

People in manual jobs, or those unemployed, may not know what services are available or what damage smoking and drinking too much are doing to their health. They may not realise that a poor diet and obesity means they are more likely to suffer from cancer, heart disease and breathing problems. People in lower skilled jobs are also more likely to suffer from violence and their children are more likely to have accidents than those of the professional classes. Unfortunately research shows a clear link between poor health and lower social class.

The homeless have least access to health care because an address is needed to register with a GP. Most homeless people do not get health care until they attend a hospital emergency department. Primary care and outreach work try to make sure more people can get health care.

Family structure

Studied ▢

Family structure impacts on access to care. A single parent may have little money so cannot afford to pay for dental treatment or eye tests for themselves. They may have no one to leave the children with if they need to go into hospital, so may be reluctant to see the doctor. A nuclear family with two parents may find paying for dental treatment less of a problem, especially if both are working. Childcare may be less of a problem with an extended family as there is always someone to look after the children, so members of an extended family may be more likely to access services. They are more likely to access services for children. Sure Start centres have been effective in improving access to health and care services for children and families.

Those living alone, especially the elderly, do not necessarily access services. They may not realise they are ill or may not have transport to get to services. Less has been done to help them access services.

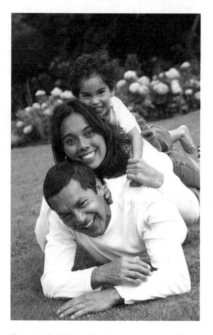

Figure 2.5 Family structure can affect access to care

Geographical location

Studied

Geographical location, where you live, impacts on access to health and social care services. In rural areas, people may travel many miles to a hospital, but those living in a city may have several nearby. In the city, people have a wider choice of doctors, dentists and other services.

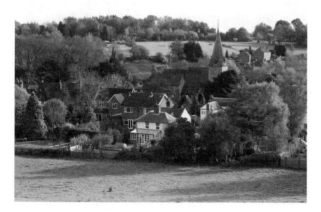

Figure 2.6 Living in a rural area can reduce access to care

How adapting services to meet the diverse needs of service users promotes equality and diversity in health and social care

Adaptations to services to meet the diverse needs of service users

We adapt services to meet individual needs based on the factors described below:

- Gender
- Sexual orientation
- Gender reassignment
- Age
- Disability
- Marriage and civil partnerships
- Pregnancy and maternity
- Race
- Religion and belief
- Social class
- Family structure
- Geographical location.

Services should be adapted to meet the diverse needs of service users, for example:

- **Access to services.** Everyone should be able to have basic health care from a GP, even if they do not have a fixed address. Travellers and the homeless have difficulty getting a GP.
- **Provision of support.** This should be available according to need, not according to where you live. Fertility treatment is available in some areas but not others.
- **Dietary requirements.** Care services now offer a choice of vegetarian or non-vegetarian meals and some vegan food is available. Halal and kosher meals are becoming more widely available in hospitals.
- **Provision of personal care.** Some individuals require help with washing and toileting. The individual's needs should be assessed.
- **Provision of prayer facilities.** Hospitals offer a multi-faith prayer room so all faiths and people of no faith can use it.

- **Access to washing and toilet facilities.** This is a basic human need. Services are adapted by allowing more space so that people with mobility issues can access the toilet and washing facilities. Doors are widened to allow wheelchair access or separate provision is made to provide these facilities.

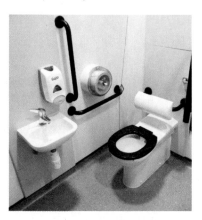

Figure 2.7 Toilet facilities for people with disabilities

- **Observing religious rituals.** All faiths and beliefs must be respected. Catholics may wish to have the last rites read to them if they are dying and may request that a priest is sent for to do this.
- **Visiting arrangements.** Visiting arrangements should be flexible for people in residential care so that family and friends can maintain contact.
- **Provision of person-centred approach.** Putting the service user at the centre and looking at their needs will ensure services are adapted to meet their needs. Examples of person-centred care are given throughout this section.
- **Same-sex carers.** Some individuals feel comfortable only with carers of the same sex. There may be cultural or religious reasons why they do not wish to have a carer of the opposite sex. Where possible their wishes should be met, but if it is not possible, the situation should be explained to them. They may be able to suggest an alternative solution.
- **Provision of opportunity and places of worship.** Hospitals already provide places of worship. Residential care may not always have space for a prayer room, but many care homes arrange for their residents to attend their preferred place of worship.
- **Mixed wards.** These cause stress for patients. The government plans to abolish them but if there is no alternative, for example in a high-dependency unit, privacy and dignity should be maintained.

- **Festivals and holy days.** These vary. Christmas, Eid, Passover and Vaishakhi are important festivals in the Christian, Islamic, Jewish and Hindu religions and service users should be equally supported in celebrating their religious festivals and holy days.

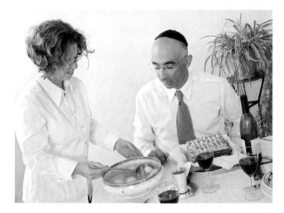

Figure 2.8 Service users should be supported to celebrate festivals and holy days

- **An awareness of practices relating to dress/clothing.** This is extremely important. Those who work in health and social care may be used to seeing people undressed, but it is not comfortable for the service user to be left half naked. In many cultures, clothing covers the head and the body from neck to foot. Sleeves are full length. It is difficult to maintain modesty and dignity in an open-backed theatre gown. The NHS are changing the design of these garments to allow for decency.
- **The level of service provided.** This promotes equality and diversity if all service users have appropriate care; for example, people with dementia require specialist care and should not be cared for by those who do not understand dementia care.
- **The provision of suitable accommodation for couples.** This promotes equality and diversity in residential care. Couples who have been married for a long time and wish to stay together when one has care needs, can now choose assisted-living housing so they can stay together.
- **Involving partners in care plans promotes equality and diversity.** A diabetic person may only be able to maintain their diet if their partner who does the cooking understands a diabetic diet.
- **The entitlement to an independent advocate.** This is especially important for people who have mental health issues or people who may have learning disabilities. Without an independent advocate, their views may be overlooked.

- **Use of appropriate language.** This promotes equality and diversity; for example, in a day centre for Asian older people, it promotes equality and diversity if carers speak some of the languages spoken by service users.
- **Use of appropriate forms of address.** This promotes equality. By addressing a person in the way they wish, carers show they respect the person's rights.
- **Acknowledging personal preferences.** This promotes equality by getting rid of favouritism. In a residential care home, some people like to watch football on television but others prefer to watch gardening. Acknowledging each person's preference and either taking turns to choose what to watch, or providing another television, shows each person is equally valued.
- **Respecting personal choices.** This shows that carers respect and value each individual. Mary might like toast in the morning but Ethel might prefer just to have porridge. By respecting personal choices, carers show they put the individual at the centre of care.

Benefits to service users of adapting services

Studied

The benefits to service users of personalised care are immense. Maintaining dignity and privacy, and making sure that service users feel safe, results in an improved quality of care and a better quality of life for all regardless of age, ability, gender or any of the factors listed earlier. Personalised and accessible care means that people keep their independence for longer, need less care input and remain active as part of a social community.

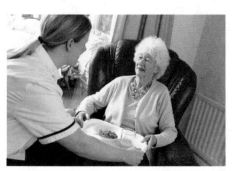

Figure 2.9 Service users will benefit from personalised care

Knowledge recap questions

1. Give five factors that may affect the care needs of individuals.

2. How may location, where you live, impact on access to health and social care services?

3. A Jehovah's Witness needs an operation. What should carers be aware of?

4. How can hospital provision show respect for religious beliefs?

5. Who may benefit from independent advocacy?

Assessment guidance for Learning aim B

Scenario

You have been volunteering at your local hospital, City Central, which takes patients from a wide range of different communities across the city. The volunteer coordinator knows you are studying health and social care and has asked you to produce a booklet to help new volunteers understand the importance of non-discriminatory practice. She has asked you to include a section on how codes of practice and legislation improve health and social care.

Some of the current volunteers read your booklet and suggest it would be good to explain and give examples of how to adapt care to meet the diverse needs of the patients admitted, basing this on at least two patients with differing needs.

You will need to describe the different needs of service users, using examples, and describe how provision could be adapted to meet their differing needs highlighted in your examples.

You will need to explain how your proposed ideas on adapting services will benefit the two service users and assess how effective these proposed changes are likely to be in meeting their diverse needs.

The volunteer coordinator asks you to present these ideas to the next intake of volunteers so you will need to prepare a presentation with notes.

2B.P3 Describe the different needs of service users in health and social care, with reference to examples

Assessor report: The command verb in the grading criteria is **describe**. The learner should give a clear description of potential individual needs related to all the factors listed in the unit content and give at least one example for each category of diverse needs. The categories are: gender, sexual orientation, gender reassignment, age, disability, marriage and civil partnerships, pregnancy and maternity, race, religion and belief, social class, family structure, geographical location. Examples should be from a range of health and social care settings so that learners can find out about the diverse needs of individuals receiving different types of service.

Learner answer

People are individuals and each person has different needs. There are different types of need. These include gender, sexual orientation, gender reassignment, age, disability, marriage and civil partnerships, pregnancy and maternity, race, religion and belief, social class, family structure, geographical location.

Assessor report: The learner has made a good start by listing the different needs of service users in health and social care. They will now need to provide a description of each of these different needs and use examples.

 Learner answer

A person may have needs according to their gender; for example, a woman may develop breast cancer and need advice about what to wear to maintain a good body image. Men sometimes develop breast cancer but their body image may be less affected by it than a woman's.

People may have needs around sexual orientation. People who are gay, lesbian, bisexual or transsexual may need advice and emotional support if they are just coming to terms with their sexuality. Some voluntary organisations provide this.

Individuals considering or going through gender reassignment may need counselling to help them come to terms with the changes and how to cope with the reactions of others.

As people age, their needs change. They may be able to manage very well while they have family and friends around, but as they grow older and their friends do too, it may be difficult for them to cope with shopping and cooking and they may need help such as Meals on Wheels to make sure they get a cooked meal.

Family structure may impact on needs. An 80-year-old person living alone may find it difficult to cope and may need help from social services in deciding whether to move into a residential home or into sheltered housing. A single parent struggling to manage may need help with budgeting and some advice on benefits from social services.

Where someone lives, geographical location, can affect their needs. Travellers who move frequently may have difficulty getting a General Practitioner and so may need to use emergency services more often. People who are homeless may also use emergency services as they cannot get a GP. For people living in the countryside, and without transport, they may need help to attend a hospital which may be many miles away. Hospital transport may be needed.

Assessor report – overall

What is good about this assessment evidence?

Each factor is described and the learner gives an example for each factor mentioned. Gender, sexual orientation, gender reassignment, age, family structure and geographical location are covered.

What could be improved about this assessment evidence?

In order to achieve 2B.P3, the learner should include the remaining factors and give an example for each. The remaining factors to cover are: disability, marriage and civil partnerships, pregnancy and maternity, race, religion and belief, and social class.

2B.P4 **Describe how health and social care provision can be adapted to meet the diverse needs of different individuals, with reference to examples**

Assessor report: The command verb in the grading criteria is **describe**. Learners should provide a clear description of how health and social care staff and settings can adapt services to meet the diverse needs of individuals. Examples are needed. Learners could either provide a brief example for each category or make reference to a couple of detailed examples.

 Learner answer

Health and social care provision can be adapted to meet the diverse needs of different individuals.

Instead of a general nurse giving advice, a breast cancer nurse specialist may offer advice on what clothing to wear to help the woman feel good about her body image.

People may have needs around sexual orientation. A survey found that lesbian and bisexual women did not attend a general clinic for sexual health screening and cervical screening because they felt their health needs were not understood. A clinic was set up to cater for their specific needs and offer screening for sexually transmitted infections, and to offer sexual health education as well as safer sex advice.

Assessor report: The learner has made a good start in describing how health and social care provision can be adapted to meet the needs of sexual orientation, providing an example of a clinic set up to cater for the specific needs of lesbian and bisexual women. The learner now needs to provide similar descriptions and examples for other needs of different individuals.

 Learner answer

Individuals considering or going through gender reassignment may be referred by their GP to a specialist clinic that deals with all aspects of gender reassignment. One example of how services have been adapted is a specialist service provided by the NHS. There are several centres but one is the Laurels Gender Identity

31

and Sexual Medicine Service which is part of Devon Partnership NHS Trust. They offer psychiatric nursing, psychotherapy, counselling and general physical monitoring. There is a regular support group and after a long process of counselling, surgery may be offered.

As people age, their needs change. Most local authorities offer specialist social services for older people and aim to increase independence, choice and control in daily life and enable older people to find out about other support services. Other services may be direct payment, home care, day care, equipment, meals at home, residential or nursing care and sheltered housing.

Family structure may impact on needs. A single parent struggling to manage may need help with budgeting and some advice on benefits. Much of this help is available in the voluntary sector as local authority social services tend to work with single parents only when children are at risk. Gingerbread, a national charity, and Netmums, an online site for all parents, provide advice for single parents.

Where someone lives – geographical location – can affect their needs. Travellers who move frequently may have difficulty getting a General Practitioner. There have been recent changes in primary care and this situation was looked at. The NHS now advise GPs that they should see members of the traveller community without an appointment.

People living in the countryside, and without transport, may need help to attend a hospital which may be many miles away. Patients who receive certain benefits are able to claim for help with travel costs. Hospitals may be able to provide non-emergency patient transport for patients with a particular medical condition which stops them using private or public transport.

Assessor report – overall

What is good about this assessment evidence?

The learner has researched this and found out specific examples of how services can be adapted across health and social care.

What could be improved about this assessment evidence?

In order to achieve 2B.P4, the learner should include the remaining factors and give an example of how services can be adapted for each. The remaining factors to cover are: disability, marriage and civil partnerships, pregnancy and maternity, race, religion and belief, and social class.

2B.M2 Explain the benefits of adapting health and social care provision to meet the diverse needs of different individuals, with reference to two selected examples

Assessor report: The command verb in the grading criteria is **explain.** Learners should provide details and give reasons for the benefits of adapting health and social care provision to meet diverse needs. They should use examples of two individuals with different needs to illustrate this.

✍ Learner answer

Mr and Mrs X are Hindu, in their 80s and have been married for over 60 years. Mr X had a stroke last year and since then has been unable to get upstairs. He has carers who come in to help him get washed and dressed in the morning as Mrs X, who is frail, is unable to manage this for him. Their grown-up daughter lives at the other end of the country and is worried about them. She wants them to come and live with her but they want to keep their independence and they do not get on with her husband. The family have considered whether Mr X should go into a residential care home but Mrs X does not want to be separated from her husband and does not want him to be in a care home as she does not think they give good care. She is also worried that they will not provide a tasty vegetarian diet for him and he will stop eating. Even with carers coming in to help, life is now getting very difficult for both of them.

In this example Mr X has needs around both age and disability while Mrs X has needs because of her age. Marriage is a factor which affects their needs, as do religion and beliefs. The social worker advising them suggests that sheltered housing may be an alternative for them. They can have what care they want and be as independent as they like. Mrs X can cook in her own flat or they can have a cooked meal in the restaurant. Help is always at hand if needed and the charges include an hour a week of cleaning so they do not have to worry about housework. Fortunately they do not have to worry about money as they have savings and their daughter and son-in-law will help them.

The benefits of this service are that they can keep independent for as long as they wish. Mr and Mrs X can still go to the temple when they wish, but they know there is always help at hand if they need it. Having their own home means they maintain dignity and privacy, but still feel safe. This results in a better quality of life for them. They are more likely to meet people and less likely to get depressed. Personalised and accessible care means that they keep their independence for longer. They may need less care input as they remain active as part of a social community. Mentally and physically they will benefit.

Assessor report: The learner has given a detailed example of how care services can be adapted to meet the needs of older people who have needs around ageing, disability and religious beliefs.

Assessor report – overall

What is good about this assessment evidence?

The learner has used a detailed case study, researched what is available and shown how care services adapt to individual needs.

What could be improved about this assessment evidence?

A second detailed example is required to achieve 2B.M2. The case should include multiple needs to ensure coverage of as many factors as possible.

2B.D2 **Assess the effectiveness of health and social care provision for different individuals with diverse needs, with reference to two selected examples**

Assessor report: The command verb in the grading criteria is **assess**. For 2B.D2, learners should extend their work for 2B.M2 to assess the usefulness (effectiveness) of this provision for individuals with diverse needs. Learners should consider the categories of needs which were used earlier in the assignment and make a judgement as to whether provision was appropriate and sufficient overall, or whether it was inappropriate or insufficient. The conclusion reached should follow on logically from the evidence presented, so if evidence shows there is enough provision, the judgement cannot be that it is insufficient.

✍ **Learner answer**

Sheltered accommodation provided an ideal solution for Mr and Mrs X because it offered the service they needed at a price they could afford, so for them it was effective at the time. There are issues around social class and how much money a person has. Mr and Mrs X were lucky that they could afford sheltered housing, but some older people who would like to live in sheltered housing and have these services cannot afford the charges. Some charities provide sheltered accommodation for certain groups in some places, but the service is not provided everywhere. Sheltered housing is effective in maintaining independence and quality of life for those who can afford it, however the service is not available to all. There is not enough of this provision at a price that all who need it can afford.

Assessor report: The learner has made a good start, with an assessment of the effectiveness of the provision of one service.

Assessor report – overall

What is good about this assessment evidence?

The learner makes a judgement that provision was appropriate but insufficient, based on evidence.

What could be improved about this assessment evidence?

A second detailed example is required and the learner should make a judgement of appropriateness and sufficiency based on the evidence presented.

Sample assignment brief 1: The importance of non-discriminatory practice in health and social care

PROGRAMME NAME	BTEC Level 2 First Award in Health and Social Care
ASSIGNMENT TITLE	The importance of non-discriminatory practice in health and social care
ASSESSMENT EVIDENCE	Booklet

This assignment will assess the following learning aim and grading criteria:

Learning aim A: Understand the importance of non-discriminatory practice in health and social care

2A.P1 Describe non-discriminatory and discriminatory practice in health and social care, using examples.

2A.P2 Describe how codes of practice and legislation promote non-discriminatory practice in health and social care.

2A.M1 Explain the importance of legislation and codes of practice in promoting non-discriminatory practice in health and social care, using examples.

2A.D1 Assess the impact of discriminatory practice for health and social care workers, with reference to selected examples.

Scenario

You have been volunteering at your local health centre, which takes patients from a wide range of different communities across the city. The volunteer coordinator knows you are studying health and social care and has asked you to produce a booklet to help new volunteers understand the importance of non-discriminatory practice. She has asked you to include a section on how codes of practice and legislation improve health and social care.

Include the following and give examples for each:

- A description of non-discriminatory and discriminatory practice
- A description of how codes of practice and current and relevant legislation promote non-discriminatory practice, explaining their importance in promoting non-discriminatory practice
- An assessment of the potential impact of discriminatory practice for health and social care workers.

Task 1

Describe discriminatory and non-discriminatory practices. Illustrate your understanding by giving examples of non-discriminatory or discriminatory practices for three of these categories:

- Examples of **discrimination** in health and social care, e.g. prejudice, stereotyping, labelling, refusal of medical treatment, offering inappropriate treatment or care, giving less time when caring for an individual than needed.

- Examples of **non-discriminatory practice** in health and social care, e.g. providing appropriate health and social care to meet the needs of individuals, adapting care to meet the diverse needs of different individuals, providing equality of access to health and social care services.

Task 2

Describe how codes of practice and legislation promote non-discriminatory practice in health and social care. Describe at least two codes of practice; these may be for either social care or health practitioners and should be the current versions of the codes. You do not need to know the complex details of these codes.

Task 3

Extend your work for Tasks 1 and 2 to explain the importance of legislation and codes of practice in promoting non-discriminatory practice in health and social care, using at least two relevant examples. Use current and relevant legislation and codes of practice. Examples may be either of non-discriminatory practice, or discriminatory practices. Highlight the respective benefits or negative consequences of each.

Task 4

Using the two examples from Task 3, assess the impact of discriminatory practice for health and social care workers.

Sample assignment brief 2: How health and social care practices can promote equality and diversity

PROGRAMME NAME	**BTEC Level 2 First Award in Health and Social Care**
ASSIGNMENT TITLE	**How health and social care practices can promote equality and diversity**
ASSESSMENT EVIDENCE	**Individual or small-group PowerPoint presentations, written reports, leaflets or handbooks.**

This assignment will assess the following learning aim and grading criteria:

Learning aim B: Explore how health and social care practices can promote equality and diversity

2B.P3 Describe the different needs of service users in health and social care, with reference to examples.

2B.P4 Describe how health and social care provision can be adapted to meet the diverse needs of different individuals, with reference to examples.

2B.M2 Explain the benefits of adapting health and social care provision to meet the diverse needs of different individuals, with reference to two selected examples.

2B.D2 Assess the effectiveness of health and social care provision for different individuals with diverse needs, with reference to two selected examples.

Scenario

You have been volunteering at your health centre, which takes patients from a wide range of different communities across the city. The volunteer coordinator knows you are studying health and social care and has asked you to produce a booklet to help new volunteers understand the importance of non-discriminatory practice. She has asked you to include a section on how codes of practice and legislation improve health and social care.

Some of the current volunteers read your booklet and suggest it would be good to explain and give examples of how to adapt care to meet the diverse needs of the patients admitted, basing this on at least two patients with differing needs.

You will need to describe the different needs of service users, using examples, and describe how provision could be adapted to meet their differing needs highlighted in your examples.

You will need to explain how your proposed ideas on adapting services will benefit the two service users and assess how effective these proposed changes are likely to be in meeting their diverse needs.

The volunteer coordinator asks you to present these ideas to the next intake of volunteers so you will need to prepare a presentation with notes.

Task 1

Give a clear description of potential individual needs related to the following categories: gender, sexual orientation, gender reassignment, age, disability, marriage and civil partnerships, pregnancy and maternity, race, religion and belief, social class, family structure and geographical location.

For each category, give at least one example. Examples should be from a range of health and social care settings so that you can find out about the diverse needs of individuals receiving different types of service.

Task 2

Describe how health and social care staff and settings can adapt services to meet the diverse needs of individuals. Use examples and either provide a brief example for each category or refer to a couple of detailed examples.

Task 3

Explain the benefits of adapting health and social care provision to meet diverse needs of individuals. Use examples of two individuals with different needs to illustrate this.

Task 4

Using your work for Task 3, assess the usefulness (effectiveness) of this provision for individuals with diverse needs. Consider the categories of needs which were used earlier in the assignment and make a judgement whether provision was appropriate and sufficient overall or whether it was inappropriate or insufficient. Make sure that the conclusion you reach follows on logically from the evidence presented, so if evidence shows there is enough provision and it works, the judgement has to be that it is sufficient, or if your evidence shows that provision is inappropriate or that it does not work, the judgement has to be that it is ineffective.

Assessment criteria

Level 2 Pass	Level 2 Merit	Level 2 Distinction
Learning aim A: Understand the importance of non-discriminatory practice in health and social care		
2A.P1 Describe non-discriminatory and discriminatory practice in health and social care, using examples.	2A.M1 Explain the importance of legislation and codes of practice in promoting non-discriminatory practice in health and social care, using examples.	2A.D1 Assess the impact of discriminatory practice for health and social care workers, with reference to selected examples.
2A.P2 Describe how codes of practice and legislation promote non-discriminatory practice in health and social care.		
Learning aim B: Explore how health and social care practices can promote equality and diversity		
2B.P3 Describe the different needs of service users in health and social care, with reference to examples.		
2B.P4 Describe how health and social care provision can be adapted to meet the diverse needs of different individuals, with reference to examples.	2B.M2 Explain the benefits of adapting health and social care provision to meet the diverse needs of different individuals, with reference to two selected examples.	2B.D2 Assess the effectiveness of health and social care provision for different individuals with diverse needs, with reference to two selected examples.

Answers: Unit 7 Knowledge recap

Learning aim A: Understand the importance of non-discriminatory practice in health and social care

1. 'Non-discriminatory practice' means:
   - not treating individuals or groups less fairly than others
   - we should treat individuals and groups fairly
   - valuing diversity, seeing differences as a positive thing
   - adapting care to meet diverse needs.

2. This is an example of discriminatory practice because it is not treating people fairly.

3. This is an example of non-discriminatory practice because it is giving each person access to information.

4. The effects of discrimination (bad practice) on service users include:
   - loss of self-esteem
   - stress
   - reluctance to seek support and treatment
   - longer waiting times for some groups.

5. The Equality Act 2010 protects people from discrimination, harassment and victimisation on the grounds of:
   - age
   - disability
   - gender reassignment
   - marriage and civil partnership
   - pregnancy and maternity
   - race
   - religion or belief
   - sex
   - sexual orientation.

6. The General Social Care Council publishes a code of conduct for employers of social care workers and one for social care workers too. The Nursing and Midwifery Council (NMC) has a code of conduct for professional nurses and midwives.

Learning aim B: Explore how health and social care practices can promote equality and diversity

1. Any five from the following:
   - gender
   - sexual orientation
   - gender reassignment
   - age
   - disability
   - marriage and civil partnership
   - pregnancy and maternity
   - race
   - religion and belief
   - social class
   - family structure
   - geographical location.

2. In rural areas, people may travel many miles to a hospital but those living in a city may have several hospitals nearby. In the city, people have a wider choice of doctors, dentists and other services.

3. Jehovah's Witnesses do not accept blood transfusions, so the operation may possibly be cancelled if a blood transfusion is required for the operation.

4. Provision of prayer facilities – hospitals offer a multi-faith prayer room so all faiths and people of no faith can use it.

5. The entitlement to an independent advocate is especially important for people who have mental health issues or people who may have learning disabilities.

Index

Index